The Language of Hospital Services in English

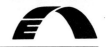

Gretchen Bloom   English For Careers

The Language of Hospital Services in English

PRENTICE HALL REGENTS, Englewood Cliffs, NJ 07632

We wish to acknowledge the generous assistance
of the following:

Georgetown University Medical Center
Manhattan Eye, Ear and Throat Hospital
Montefiore Hospital and Medical Center
The New York Hospital—Cornell Medical Center

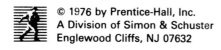

Printed in the United States of America

10 9 8 7 6 5 4 3 2 1

ISBN   0-13-523176-0   01

Prentice-Hall International (UK) Limited, London
Prentice-Hall of Australia Pty. Limited, Sydney
Prentice-Hall Canada Inc., Toronto
Prentice-Hall Hispanoamericana, S.A., Mexico
Prentice-Hall of India Private Limited, New Delhi
Prentice-Hall of Japan, Inc., Tokyo
Simon & Schuster Asia Pte. Ltd., Singapore
Editora Prentice-Hall do Brasil, Ltda., Rio de Janeiro

TABLE OF CONTENTS

FOREWORD

This book is one of a series of texts called *English for Careers*. The series is intended to introduce students of English as a foreign language to the language of different professional and vocational fields. The career areas that are covered are those in which English is widely used throughout the world, such as air travel, computer programming, the petroleum industry, international banking, and so on.

Each book in the series serves several purposes. The first is to give the student an introduction to the particular vocational area in which he or she is involved. The duties of different kinds of jobs are discussed, as well as the problems that might be encountered at work. In this particular book, *The Language of Hospital Services in English*, the jobs of the personnel who staff a hospital are discussed. Medical jobs are included, but equally important are the jobs performed by the various technical, administrative, and other kinds of personnel essential to the operation of a hospital. The book is not intended as a detailed training manual, but rather as a broad introduction both to the occupations and the problems involved in this kind of work.

American hospitals have been used as models in this book. However, the manner in which American hospitals function is basically the same in hospitals throughout the world.

From the point of view of teaching English as a foreign language, these books are intended for a student at the high intermediate or the advanced level. In other words, the student who uses these books should be acquainted with most of the structural patterns of English. His principal goals as a learner should be mastering vocabulary, using the various patterns in a normal mixture, and improving his ability to communicate in English.

These books address themselves to all of these needs. Each unit begins with a glossary of special terms in which words and expressions used in the vocational areas being discussed are defined. This glossary is followed by a vocabulary study that tests the student's comprehension of the special terms and gives practice in their use. In the reading, these terms are used again within a contextual frame of reference. Each reading is followed by questions for comprehension and discussion. They give the student the opportunity to use in a communicative situation both the vocabulary items and the structural patterns that have occurred in the reading.

Each unit ends with an exercise or exercises, some of which pose problems that might occur if the student were working at the job. He might, for instance, be asked to fill out forms that are used on the job; or he might have to make up short dialogues that involve human problems and situations that arise in connection with the job. In doing these exercises, he will also practice the specialized vocational vocabulary and other new words, as well as the structural patterns that are used with them.

A great deal of successful language learning comes from experiences in which the learning is largely unconscious. In offering these books, it is hoped that the student's interest in his chosen field will increase his ability to communicate more effectively in English.

The author of this book wishes to express her appreciation to the staff at Georgetown University Hospital in Washington, D.C. for their cooperation in making available much of the material on which this book is based.

GRETCHEN BLOOM
Washington, D.C.

UNIT ONE
THE MODERN HOSPITAL:
AN OVERVIEW

Special Terms

Hospital: An institution in which sick or injured persons are given medical or surgical treatment. The first hospitals were no more than rest houses for the sick. Modern hospitals provide a variety of services.

Patient: A sick or injured person who makes use of the medical services offered by the hospital.

Community Hospital: The most common type of hospital. It offers general, short-term care to *acutely* or severely ill patients. It differs from specialized hospitals and hospitals that provide long-term care for *chronic* or recurrent conditions.

Voluntary Hospital: A private, nonprofit hospital that is financed by private contributions and sometimes by government grants. Most hospitals in the United States are voluntary hospitals.

Proprietary Hospital: A hospital that is run to make a profit.

Health Insurance: A form of protection against unexpected high medical costs. The purchaser makes regular payments called *premiums* to an insurance company. In return, he or she expects the insurance company to pay a percentage of medical expenses. *Blue Cross* and *Blue Shield* are very popular private plans in the United States. *Medicare* and *Medicaid* are sponsored by the United States government at a nominal cost to the insured.

Hospital Board: The policy-making body for the hospital. It is also known as the *board of directors* or *board of trustees*. They hire the

1

hospital administrator, approve the medical staff, and make the major decisions about the services offered by the hospital. Their decisions are based on the advice of a number of hospital committees.

Hospital Administrator: The person in charge of running a hospital. Hired by the board of directors, this individual is responsible for coordinating the various services provided by the hospital.

Medical Director: The physician responsible for the medical services in the hospital. He or she is usually appointed by the board and advised by members of the medical staff.

Medical Advisory Board: A *standing*, or permanent, *committee* that advises the hospital board on general medical policies. This group is also referred to as the *joint conference committee.*

Accredited: Certified or approved by the Joint Commission on Accreditation of Hospitals. All hospitals must meet certain standards of health care before they can be officially accredited.

Ladies' Auxiliary: A group of volunteers who support the hospital. They raise funds and work without pay.

Vocabulary Practice

1. What is the purpose of a *hospital?*

2. What is the name given to a sick or injured person who makes use of a hospital?

3. Define the term *community hospital.*

4. What is meant by *acute* illness? *Chronic* illness?

5. Does a *community hospital* usually accept patients who need long-term care?

6. What is the difference between a *voluntary hospital* and a *proprietary hospital?*

7. What is *health insurance?* What is a *premium?*

8. Give an example of a private *health insurance* plan and a government-sponsored plan.

9. What is the governing body of a hospital called? Give two names.

10. Who is the person responsible for running a hospital?

11. Who oversees the medical services offered by a hospital?

12. What does the *medical advisory board* do?

13. What is another name for the *medical advisory board?*

14. What is a *standing* committee?

15. What does it mean for a hospital to be *accredited?*

16. What does the *ladies' auxiliary* do?

The Modern Hospital: An Overview

The modern *hospital* is one of many institutions responsible for providing health care to the sick and injured, but it is probably the most familiar and certainly the most complex. It hardly resembles the earlier institutions that were also known as hospitals. Advances in medical science have created a virtual revolution in the health services field. The quality of care available to *patients* has improved; the need for personnel trained in the health professions has grown; and the variety of ways for people to work with the sick and injured has increased. Years ago, an individual had the choice of becoming a doctor, a dentist, or a hospital administrator. Today, he or she can choose from hundreds of health-related professions.

Many of these personnel, trained in a variety of fields, are needed to staff a modern hospital to provide adequate patient care. Most people forget that patients have many kinds of needs. They must be fed; their medical records must be kept; the floors must be kept clean;

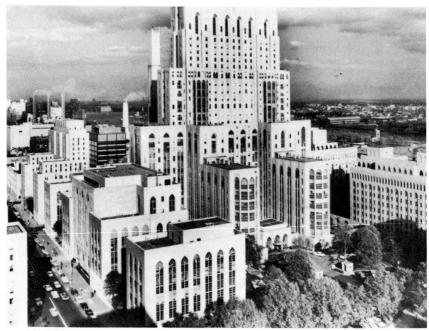

A modern hospital. (Courtesy The New York Hospital—Cornell Medical Center)

and the laundry must be washed. In addition, employees have to be hired and equipment has to be purchased. These are some of the countless tasks that must be performed efficiently and properly by the hospital staff.

Hospitals were not always so complex. In India, hospitals existed as early as the fourth century B.C. But they were really only rest houses where the sick remained until they either recovered or died. In ancient Greece and Rome, temples were often used as hospitals. These early hospitals were clean, pleasant places, but they did not pay much attention to the body. The name hospital, in fact, is derived from the Latin word *hospitium*, which means "a place where guests are received." The English words *hotel* and *hostel* are derived from this same root.

The Church assumed the primary responsibility for the care of the sick during the Middle Ages. Hospitals continued to be used as rest houses, but they gradually acquired a bad reputation. They became known as places of filth and death, to be avoided at all costs. It is no wonder that early American settlers in the New World did not want to establish hospitals. It was not until 1713 that William Penn founded the first community hospital in the colonies in Philadelphia.

During the nineteenth century, medical advances changed all this. Louis Pasteur developed his germ theory, and Florence Nightingale made nursing a respectable profession. Since then, the number of hospitals has grown dramatically in the world. By 1873, in the United States alone, there were nearly 200 hospitals. Today, there are more than 7,000.

There are many different kinds of hospitals. The most common is the general or *community hospital*. It treats patients of all ages and numerous illnesses and injuries. Most patients have *acute* problems and usually stay less than a week.

Other hospitals provide more specialized care. Some treat patients with *chronic* illnesses and offer facilities for long-term care. Others take patients of only one age group, such as children, or patients with one particular illness, such as tuberculosis.

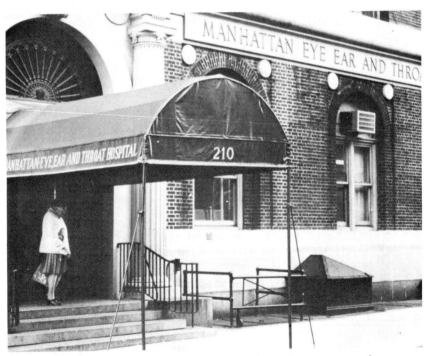

Manhattan Eye, Ear and Throat Hospital, a voluntary, nonprofit, specialty hospital. (Courtesy Manhattan Eye, Ear and Throat Hospital)

Hospitals can also be categorized according to the nature of their financial support. Most hospitals in the world are financed by the government of the country in which they are located. This is not true in the United States, where only military hospitals and some other specialized institutions are run by federal, state, or local government. Here hospitals tend to be private, nonprofit institutions. These *voluntary hospitals* are usually associated with universities or religious groups. Some of their operating expenses may be paid for by government grants. Most of their revenues, however, must come from private endowments and gifts.

Operating a hospital has become extremely costly. As a result, patients often cannot afford to pay these expenses. Fortunately, different kinds of health insurance are available. In the United States, the federal government assists those over 65 years of age with a health plan called *Medicare*. Those under 65 who are unable to pay insurance *premiums* are eligible for *Medicaid* assistance. Most other people are protected by private insurance plans. Two of the most popular of these are *Blue Cross* and *Blue Shield*.

A third kind of hospital, in addition to government-financed and nonprofit, is the *proprietary hospital*. This kind of hospital is private and is run to make a profit. It is usually small and located where there are no other adequate health care facilities.

Most hospitals are governed by a *hospital board*, which is also known as the *board of directors* or *board of trustees*. This board is made up of a variety of citizens of the community who serve on a voluntary, nonpaid basis. The board must make sure that the hospital provides efficient and economical health care to its patients. It is also responsible for maintaining adequate medical standards. To achieve this, the board hires a *hospital administrator* to run the hospital and a *medical director* to oversee the medical staff.

A series of permanent or standing committees meets on a regular basis and advises the hospital board. The most important of these committees is the *medical advisory board*, also known as the *joint conference committee*. This committee is made up of the medical director, selected staff physicians who are their department heads, and the hospital administrator. It advises the board on general medical matters and reviews the performance of the doctors. Other standing committees include finance, education, public relations, personnel, long-term planning, buildings-and-grounds, and nominating committees.

Many hospitals are also linked to the community through their volunteer programs. These are still frequently referred to as *ladies' auxiliaries*, because most of their volunteers have been women. Some volunteers help by soliciting community support for hospitals. Others actually work in the hospitals, helping to serve food trays or to select books for patients from the library cart. Some volunteers may even be involved in occupational therapy or perhaps in other semi-medical capacities. Many hospital gift shops are run by ladies' auxiliaries. Other kinds of volunteers include teenagers who are often known as *candy stripers*. They are called this because they wear pink-and-white striped uniforms to distinguish themselves from the nurses.

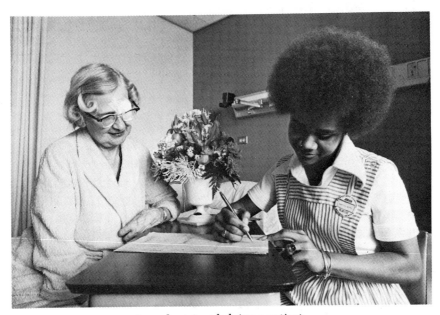

A candy striper helping a patient.
(Courtesy Montefiore Hospital and Medical Center)

The American Hospital Association has done much to improve the standards of hospital care in the United States. Founded in 1899, the AHA holds annual meetings, maintains a library service, and publishes materials to help hospitals improve their care. One of the goals of the AHA has been to encourage more hospitals to seek accreditation. Most hospitals in the United States now are *accredited* by the Joint Commission on Accreditation of Hospitals. A hospital must offer two essential services before it can be accredited. It must have both an organized medical staff that provides responsible medical care and a staff of licensed, registered nurses on duty at all times. The following support facilities must also be available: a dietary department, a medical records division, a pharmacy, a pathology department, a radiology department, an emergency care unit, and a medical library. It is the responsibility of the board of directors to assure that these facilities are provided.

The following description of the organizational structure of Georgetown University Hospital in Washington, D. C. may help to illustrate how a modern hospital functions.

Georgetown University Hospital offers a variety of medical facilities through its many clinical departments. There are, for example, departments of general medicine, psychiatry, anesthesia, pediatrics, surgery, pathology, radiation therapy, neurology, ophthalmology, radiology, emergency service, physical medicine and rehabilitation, oral surgery, ambulatory care, laboratories, and obstetrics and gynecology. Each of these departments is run by a chairman who is reponsible to the medical director.

The hospital administrator at Georgetown University Hospital handles the various administrative services that support the medical staff. The administrator is assisted by an associate administrator, five assistant administrators, and several administrative assistants. The five assistant administrators are in charge of the five service areas: nursing, financial affairs, materials management, hospital services, and professional services.

Both the medical director and the hospital administrator are directly responsible to the chancellor for medical center affairs. The chancellor is in turn responsible to the university president, who is appointed by the board of directors for the university. The chancellor for medical center affairs must also concern himself with the schools of medicine, dentistry, and nursing.

The subsequent units in this book will examine the various services offered by most hospitals in greater detail. Attention will be paid to administrative, technical, and institutional facilities, as well as the medical services.

Discussion

1. What complex yet familiar institution provides health care to the sick and injured?

2. What have been some of the results of recent advances in medical science?

3. How did the first hospitals differ from modern hospitals?

4. Describe a community hospital. What kind of care does it offer?

5. How are most hospitals in the world financed?

6. How are most hospitals in the United States financed?

7. With hospital costs as high as they are, how do patients manage to pay their bills?

8. Name two of the most popular private health insurance plans in the United States. How do they differ from Medicare? From Medicaid?

9. Define the duties of the hospital board.

10. What two employees does the hospital board usually hire? What do they do?

11. What is the medical advisory board? Name some of the other standing committees found in most hospitals.

12. Where does the term *candy stripers* come from?

13. How do volunteers help in the hospital?

14. What are the purposes of the American Hospital Association?

15. What does the Joint Commission on Accreditation of Hospitals do?

16. What are some of the services that must be provided by a hospital in addition to medical services?

Review

A. Try to imagine all the needs you would have as a patient in a hospital. What services would you expect the hospital to provide to meet those needs?

B. Write an agenda for a possible hospital board meeting, imagining a number of issues that might realistically be discussed.

UNIT TWO
THE ADMINISTRATION OF A
MODERN HOSPITAL

Special Terms

Hospital Administrator: The chief executive officer of the hospital. He or she is responsible for seeing that all of the services required by the hospital are provided. The hospital administrator must also make sure the hospital is run efficiently.

Associate/Assistant Administrators: Administrators who are trained in hospital administration but lack the experience to assume the top position. They must work first as associate or assistant administrators.

Administrative Assistant: Assists with various routine administrative tasks.

Medical Record: A permanent document on which everything relating to a patient's medical diagnosis and treatment during his hospital stay is recorded.

Controller/Business Manager: Manages the hospital's business office. He or she is also responsible for the hospital's finances. The word *controller* is used when the person advises the administrator on financial policy. The term *business manager* applies when the person simply manages the office.

Accountant: Maintains financial records and statistical reports. He or she works in the business office.

Credit Manager: Handles the hospital's credit and collection activities. This person also works in the business office.

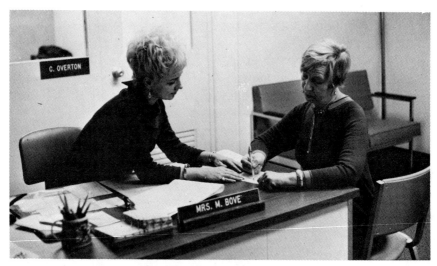

An admitting officer admitting a patient.
(Courtesy Montefiore Hospital and Medical Center)

Admitting Officer: Responsible for *admitting* or checking in patients on arrival and *discharging* or checking out patients as they leave. The admitting officer works in the business office.

Personnel Office: The office concerned with hiring and firing employees. It also makes sure that working conditions are acceptable.

Public Relations Department: A division of the hospital that must establish and maintain a good public image for the hospital.

Vocabulary Practice

1. What is the chief executive officer of a hospital called?

2. What is the difference between an *associate administrator* and an *administrative assistant?*

3. When a patient arrives at the hospital to check in, which hospital employee helps him with the procedures?

4. What word means checking patients out of a hospital?

5. Which title involves greater responsibility, *controller* or *business manager?*

6. What does an *accountant* do?

7. Whom does the *credit manager* work for?

8. What is a *medical record?*

9. What office is responsible for seeing that the hospital staff has acceptable working conditions?

10. What does the *public relations department* do?

The Administration of a Modern Hospital

The administrative task of running a modern hospital can be very complex. After all, a hospital is a health care agency, an eating establishment, a hotel, a social service and educational institution, and an office building. It must operate most of its departments 24 hours a day, 7 days a week. As a result, many different kinds of personnel are involved in running it.

All hospitals try to provide essential health services to those who need them. But most hospitals do not try to profit from their services. Because of this, hospital boards must try to raise part of the money needed to run the hospitals.

Most hospitals do not have a totally unified bureaucratic structure. This is a result of the autonomy of the medical staff. Thus, the *hospital administrator* does not have the power to manage all the parts of his organization. It is therefore essential that the board of directors hire an administrator who is able to work effectively within his established limits.

The hospital administrator serves as the chief executive officer. This person must make sure that medical and nonmedical departments function efficiently for the well-being of the patients. He or she must be healthy, energetic, and able to work under pressure. In addition, he or she must be a skillful diplomat and should enjoy working with people.

In the United States, there is a professional society for hospital

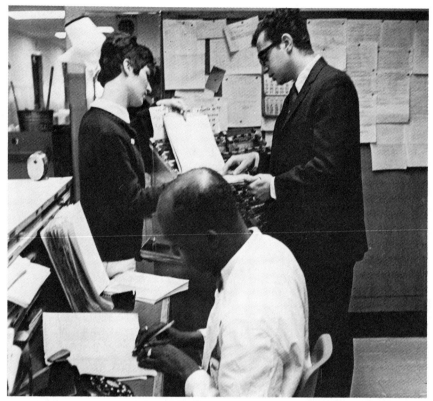

A hospital administrator at work.
(Courtesy Montefiore Hospital and Medical Center)

administrators and others who work in health care administration. It is called the American College of Hospital Administrators, ACHA for short. It was founded in 1933. Its purposes are to improve hospital administration by providing opportunities for continuing education, to publish materials that will keep administrators aware of new developments in the field, and to recognize outstanding service in the field.

As the hospital has become more complex, the administrator's role has become more challenging. As a result, the title has been changed in many areas to that of director, executive director, executive vice-president, or even president of the hospital. Because the administrator's staff often has increased in size, he can rely on the staff to perform many daily administrative tasks. This can leave the administrator free to work toward providing better health services to the community.

A hospital administrator obviously cannot perform all of the administrative tasks in a hospital. He or she is assisted by a staff of associate and assistant administrators and *administrative assistants*. At Georgetown University Hospital, as we have said, each of five assistant administrators is responsible for a major administrative area. One associate administrator works as a deputy to the administrator. These assistants in turn work closely with the business office and the public relations office.

Because most hospitals are large and complex, the administrator probably never meets most of the hospital personnel. But he is responsible for the hospital's operation and must therefore make sure that the staff is competent.

The patient who checks into a hospital probably is not aware of all of the various services he may receive during his stay. He does expect, however, to be able to receive whatever medical attention he needs. To assure that this is possible, the hospital must have a qualified administrative staff. For example, a patient assumes that someone will help him with the admitting procedures when he arrives. He also assumes that someone will show him to his room as quickly as possible. These are the duties of the *admitting officer*, who works in the business office. This person is also responsible for discharging patients at the end of their stay. Because the admitting officer is often the first hospital employee the patient deals with, he or she is generally friendly and efficient.

The business office is usually run by a *controller* or *business manager*. The business manager's job is a critical one. He is responsible for maintaining business efficiency and managing finances wisely. His responsibilities include receiving and depositing all monies, approving payments of salaries and other expenditures, and maintaining records of all incoming and outgoing transactions.

Of course, the business manager cannot perform his functions alone. An *accountant* usually helps him with financial reports. A *credit manager* usually supervises the hospital's credit and collection activities. He also helps patients to work out their payment arrangements. A cashier receives the payments. The business office is also staffed by a number of secretaries, clerks, and receptionists. They handle the necessary typing, bookkeeping, and filing; the mail and messenger services; and the telephone switchboard.

Another branch of the business office is the medical records division. A complete *medical record* must be kept on every patient. This medical record is a permanent document. It gives a complete history of all that is done for the patient during his hospital stay. It

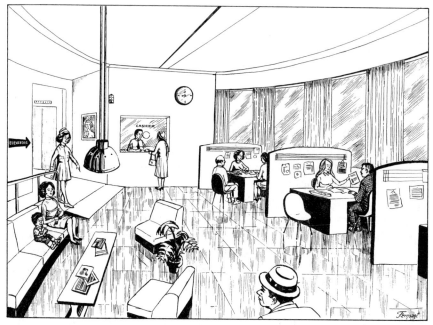

The business office of a hospital.

includes at least the following information: how the patient's condition was noticed and diagnosed; how the condition was treated; and how the patient responded to the treatment. Most hospitals have a staff of medical records technicians and librarians who maintain these important documents. Their work is supervised by a medical records administrator. A medical records employee must be orderly and accurate. In addition, medical records must be kept confidential, and this requires a strong sense of responsibility and discretion.

Another division of the business office is the *personnel office*. Someone must hire and fire hospital employees, and this is the job of the *personnel director*. To do his job well, he must know the duties of all the jobs in the hospital. He must also know the qualifications required to perform these duties. The personnel director must also assure the employees of good working conditions and answer any complaints about them. It is extremely important for the staff to have fair salaries, tolerable work schedules, adequate sick leave policies, and a good working environment. Each of these helps employees to function more efficiently.

Every hospital is interested in establishing and maintaining a good public image of itself. This is extremely important, especially if the hospital depends on the community for its financial support. To promote this image, a public relations department develops brochures and booklets to help explain the hospital's goals and services. There may also be a hospital magazine. Guides may offer regular tours of the hospital, and there may even be periodic open house events.

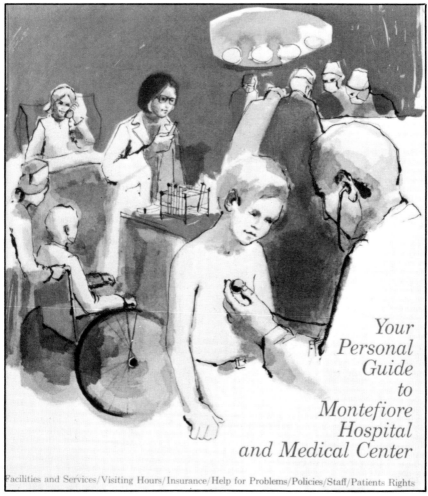

Your
Personal
Guide
to
Montefiore
Hospital
and Medical Center

Facilities and Services/Visiting Hours/Insurance/Help for Problems/Policies/Staff/Patients Rights

The cover of a brochure created by a hospital for its patients.
(Courtesy Montefiore Hospital and Medical Center)

Administrative personnel in a hospital do not have the same qualifications as the medical staff. Many people in administrative positions—such as accountants or librarians—only need training in their field. Of course, some people do need prior experience in a medical environment. Whatever the job, however, the basic goal of all hospital personnel is providing efficient care to the patients. And it must always be remembered that medical treatment is not the only kind of care that helps a patient toward recovery.

Discussion

1. How is a hospital complex?

2. What does the hospital administrator's job involve?

3. What personal qualities should a hospital administrator have?

4. What does ACHA stand for? What are its purposes?

5. How has the administrator's role changed in recent years?

6. Does the administrator have a large staff or a small one? Why?

7. Does the administrator know all of his employees?

8. Whom is a patient more likely to meet, the administrator or a member of his or her staff?

9. Is the medical staff the only staff that provides services essential to a patient's speedy recovery?

10. What does an admitting officer do?

11. Who is the director of the business office?

12. Which is more important for the business manager, to be able to deal with people or with finances?

13. Name some of the other employees in the business office. What do they do?

14. What information does a medical record contain?

15. Why must the personnel director understand the duties of all the different jobs in the hospital?

16. Why is it important for a hospital to have a good public image?

17. What working conditions are important to the hospital staff?

18. How does the public relations department create a good public image for the hospital?

19. Do the administrative personnel in a hospital need a medical background?

Review

A. You are a hospital administrator. Your personnel director reports to you that a number of nurses have complained about unfair working hours. What is your next step in resolving this complaint?

B. Prepare the following admitting form for a hospital. Help someone else fill it out as though you were an admitting officer.

NAME						JO. NO.		HISTORY NO.	
ROOM NO.	BED NO	ROOM TEL. NO	HOSP. SERV	ADMIT DATE		ADMIT TIME		DISCHARGE DATE	
ADDRESS									
BIRTH DATE		AGE	SEX	MAR	RELIGION	NEXT OF KIN			
HOME PHONE			BUSINESS PHONE			ATTENDING PHYSICIAN			
DIAGNOSIS								DIAGNOSIS CODE	

C. What kind of public relations techniques are used by the hospital in your community? Create a brochure for your hospital.

D. Complete the following sentences by filling in the blanks with the appropriate words or phrases.

1. The hospital administrator is assisted in his or her job by a number of _____ administrators.

2. The United States professional society called _____ _____ recognizes outstanding service in the field of hospital administration.

3. A patient is discharged from the hospital by the _____ _____.

4. The hospital accountant works in the _____ office.

5. A _____ gives a complete history of all that is done for a patient during his hospital stay.

6. The _____ is responsible for hiring and firing employees.

7. A hospital magazine may be published by the _____ department.

8. A hospital must operate most of its departments _____ hours a day, _____ days a week.

9. A hospital administrator might also be called a(n) _____ _____.

10. Another name for a hospital business manager is a(n) _____ _____.

UNIT THREE
BEHIND THE SCENES:
INSTITUTIONAL SERVICES

Special Terms

Purchasing Agent: Buys equipment and supplies for the hospital. He or she works in the business office.

Executive Housekeeper: Oversees a large staff of *janitors* and *maids* who keep the hospital clean. A janitor is male and a maid is female.

Chief Engineer: In charge of maintaining the equipment, buildings, and grounds of the hospital. He is helped by a large staff of plumbers, carpenters, electricians, and maintenance personnel.

Dietitian (or Dietician): A person who is trained in nutrition. A hospital employs a dietitian to plan meals for patients and employees.

Social Worker: An employee who assists patients with the transition back to the home environment. He or she works in the social services unit.

Medical Librarian: The employee trained in library science who maintains the hospital library. The library may be oriented toward the needs of the professional staff, or the library's facilities may be directed primarily toward the patients.

Chaplain: Representative of a religious faith who gives counsel and support to patients. Many hospitals have a *chapel* for religious services and for prayer.

Vocabulary Practice

1. What does a *purchasing agent* do?

2. Who is responsible for cleanliness in a hospital?

3. What is a *janitor*? A *maid*?

4. Who are some of the maintenance personnel who work for the *chief engineer*?

5. Who plans the food in a hospital?

6. What training must a *dietitian* have?

7. What does the *medical librarian* do?

8. Which employee assists patients with the transition back to the home environment?

9. What is the function of the *chaplain*?

Behind the Scenes: Institutional Services

In addition to the business and administrative aspects of managing a hospital, many other tasks must be accomplished behind the scenes in order for patients to receive proper care. None of these tasks directly affects the medical treatment offered to the patients. However, all of them are crucial to providing adequate medical care. For example, vast quantities of equipment and supplies are used in a hospital and must be replenished on a regular basis. Therefore, the hospital employs a *purchasing agent* to communicate with suppliers. He must be familiar with the thousands of goods and services that a hospital uses. He must also be an astute shopper.

When supplies are delivered, they are usually received by a stockroom manager or by a storekeeper working under the purchasing agent's direction. This storekeeper helps with the record keeping. He also helps to handle and store all the equipment.

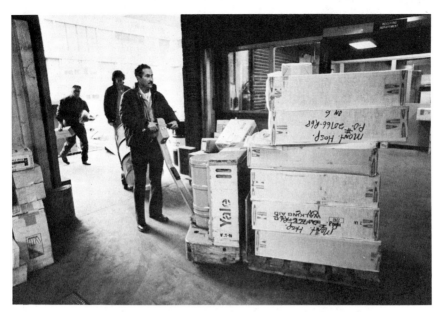

Supplies being delivered to the stockroom of a hospital.
(Courtesy Montefiore Hospital and Medical Center)

Cleanliness must be maintained throughout a hospital in order to avoid the spread of infection. An *executive housekeeper* directs a large staff of *janitors* and *maids*. They wash windows, scrub floors, mend bedclothes, and clean bathrooms. They may also take care of the laundry, although many hospitals have separate laundry departments. This is done because numerous loads of bed linen, hospital gowns, and so forth have to be washed daily.

The *chief engineer* and his maintenance staff must keep all buildings and equipment in working order. They must also maintain neat and attractive grounds. Of course, it is vital that all equipment be operative at all times. The maintenance staff may include a plumber, who is responsible for all water systems; an electrician, who maintains the wiring; a carpenter, who makes repairs when they are needed; a mason; a painter; and a groundskeeper. These employees must be skilled in their area of specialty, but prior experience in hospitals is not needed. Incidentally, all hospitals have emergency power sources. The electrician is responsible for the maintenance of these power sources. They must constantly be kept ready.

Whenever hospital remodeling or expansion is planned, the chief engineer is usually called upon for advice. Once construction is under

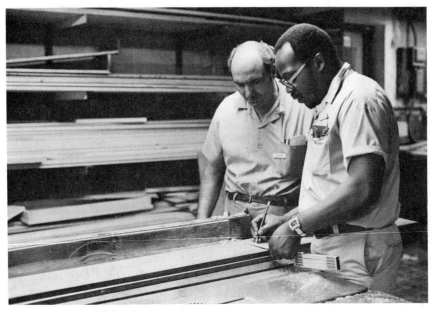

Hospital carpenters. (Courtesy Montefiore Hospital and Medical Center)

way, he often represents the administration when dealing with the various building contractors.

A patient is likely to recover more quickly from an illness or injury if he is well-nourished. It is the responsibility of the *dietitian* working on the hospital staff to see that this is the case. She has been trained to prepare wholesome meals and different kinds of diets. She confers with each patient's physician to learn the patient's special food needs, and she also advises patients on a proper diet and eating habits before they go home.

Since most patients are unable to leave their beds while they are in the hospital, a staff of kitchen attendants delivers and serves the meals to the patients' rooms. The kitchen staff usually makes special efforts to ensure that the food arrives fresh and hot. This staff is also responsible for providing food service for the hospital personnel. They usually eat in a hospital cafeteria. Visitors are often allowed to take advantage of the cafeteria.

Patients are more than statistics or case histories; they are human beings, and a good hospital treats them as human beings. An illness or injury and a period of convalescence often can be emotionally disturbing to a patient. Stress can make recovery more difficult. The hospital *social worker* is available to provide support during this important period. Patience and sympathy go hand in hand with this kind of work. The patient who responds best to medical treatment is usually the one who has been helped to relax.

Hospitals have tried very hard in recent years to discharge patients as quickly as possible and get them back into familiar surroundings. The social worker is an important aid in this kind of transition. The *psychiatric social worker* performs a similar function, but he or she usually helps people who are more acutely disturbed. The psychiatric social worker usually works closely with the staff of the mental health division of a hospital.

Still other facilities are maintained within most hospitals for the benefit of the patients, their visitors, and the staff. There is usually a library. The kind of library service that is maintained by the hospital depends on several factors: the kinds of illness that are treated, whether the hospital conducts research and training, whether a medical or nursing school is associated with the hospital, and whether the library exists primarily for the patients or for the medical staff. The *medical librarian* is responsible for the journals, books, monographs, and so on that are needed by the users of the library. The librarian should establish a book cart service for bedridden patients and create programs for those patients who are able to move about. He may also be called upon to locate information or to prepare a bibliography on a particular subject.

Most hospitals have a gift shop in the main lobby that sells newspapers, candies, and other items; it is often run by volunteers. There may also be a snack bar for visitors. A *chapel* with *chaplains* from several different religious backgrounds is common as well. All of these institutional services and facilities can make a patient's stay more pleasant and help him recover quickly.

Discussion

1. What are some of the tasks that must be accomplished behind the scenes in a hospital in addition to administrative functions?

2. What employee is responsible for buying the vast quantity of equipment and supplies used by a hospital?

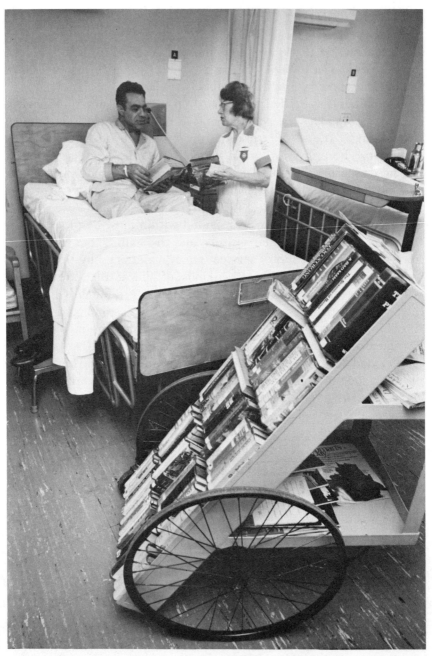

A volunteer helping a patient choose a book. Note the bookcart in the foreground.
(Courtesy Montefiore Hospital and Medical Center)

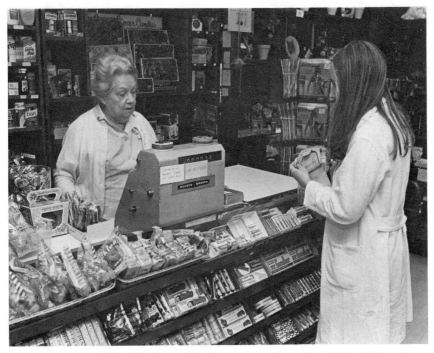

A gift shop in a hospital. (Courtesy Georgetown University Medical Center)

3. Who assists a purchasing agent?

4. Why is cleanliness especially important in a hospital?

5. Who supervises the janitors, maids, and other cleaning staff?

6. Who repairs a broken wash basin? A broken door?

7. What does a groundskeeper do?

8. Is the chief engineer usually involved if remodeling is done at the hospital? In what way?

9. Why is an adequate diet so important, especially for someone recuperating from an illness?

10. What food services must be offered in a hospital? How are most patients fed? What about hospital employees?

11. What is the purpose of the social worker?

12. Why do you think hospitals are encouraging patients to go home as soon as possible after an illness?

13. What is the difference between a social worker and a psychiatric social worker?

14. What determines the kind of library facilities that a hospital maintains?

15. How do patients confined to their beds make use of the library?

16. Who often runs the hospital gift shop?

17. How do you think a chaplain can be helpful to a sick person?

Review

A. It is imperative that the equipment in a hospital be in good working condition at all times. Describe what problems might develop if the electricity were to fail.

B. Plan a day's menus for a ward of recovering patients. Remember that patients have different needs, which depend on their conditions, and different tastes, so be sure to include a variety of choices.

C. You are the hospital social worker. Imagine that a friend of yours is a hospital patient. Try to find out all you can about his concerns, and offer any support that you feel will help.

D. Match the following terms in the left column with the most suitable definition in the right column. Only one definition is appropriate for each term.

_____ Purchasing Agent   1. Delivers meals to patients' rooms.

_____ Janitor   2. Buys supplies for the hospital.

_____ Plumber   3. Offers religious support to patients.

_____ Dietitian   4. Helps patients readjust to normal life.

_____ Social Worker   5. May work in a hospital gift shop.

_____ Librarian   6. Fixes broken water pipes.

_____ Chaplain   7. Cleans floors and washes windows.

_____ Chief Engineer   8. Plans nourishing meals for patients.

_____ Volunteer   9. Provides book cart service.

_____ Kitchen Attendant   10. Consulted about hospital remodeling.

UNIT FOUR
THE MEDICAL STAFF

Special Terms

Physician: Another name for a doctor of medicine. A physician is trained in the *practice* of medicine, the "healing art."

To Practice Medicine: To *diagnose* and *treat* patients for illness and injury, and to offer advice that will prevent further illness and injury. In the United States, a physician must be *licensed* by his or her state before being allowed to practice medicine.

Fee: The payment received by a physician from a patient for medical services. Most physicians do not receive salaries from a hospital. They simply make use of its facilities and are paid separately by the patients.

Medical Director: Chief physician in the hospital responsible for the medical staff; sometimes referred to as the *chief of staff*.

Medical Advisory Board: A committee comprised of the medical director, the hospital administrator, and selected physicians. It advises the hospital board on medical policies and reviews the performance of physicians. This committee is also known as the *joint conference committee*.

Negligence: Causing harm to a patient through carelessness.

Malpractice: Practicing medicine without a license, or causing harm to a patient by following poor medical practices. Negligence can be considered a form of malpractice.

Intern: A student doctor who has just received his medical degree. Most medical students spend one or two years as interns in a hospital. They work in various departments before getting their license to practice.

Resident: A medical student who is specializing in one field of medicine. Before being licensed in a specialty, a medical student spends two to four years as a resident physician in an accredited hospital working within that specialty. This period of time is called the *residency.*

Case: Another name for *patient.* Each patient is considered a medical case to be diagnosed and treated.

Diagnosis: Examination of a patient to determine the cause of illness. The verb form is *to diagnose.* Once the cause has been determined, an appropriate *treatment* can be suggested.

Vocabulary Practice

1. What is another name for a doctor?

2. What does *practicing medicine* involve?

3. What legal requirement must physicians meet in most states in the United States before they are allowed to practice?

4. Most physicians are not paid a salary by the hospital in which they work. How are they paid? What is this payment called?

5. What are the responsibilities of the *medical director?*

6. What is another name for the medical director?

7. What is the purpose of the *joint conference committee?* Who makes up the committee?

8. Define *negligence* and *malpractice.*

9. Most student doctors spend a year or two following the completion of their academic work rotating throughout the various medical departments in the hospital. What are they called during this period?

10. What is the purpose of a period of *residency*?

11. What is another way of referring to a patient?

12. Which comes first, *diagnosis* or *treatment*?

The Medical Staff

Since the purpose of a hospital is to care for persons who are sick or injured, the medical staff of a hospital is essential. Without doctors, a hospital could not treat patients, and there would be no reason to offer any of the other hospital services. As a matter of fact, most people think *only* of the medical staff when they think of a hospital. They forget that other personnel are necessary to the successful operation of a hospital.

Doctors belong to one of the oldest professions known to man, that of medicine. Men have dedicated themselves to the healing art—as medicine is often called—since the beginning of history. It is a very rewarding profession, but it requires a great deal of dedication. It also demands a willingness to assume responsibility for life and death.

Anyone who becomes a *physician*—another name for a doctor of medicine—has already demonstrated this dedication. He has completed at least eight years of training following high school, and between two and seven additional years if he has chosen to specialize in one particular field.

The physicians who *practice medicine* in a hospital are not usually hired by the hospital. The chief pathologist, who is in charge of the laboratory, is one exception. Most physicians have private practices. They simply make use of the hospital's facilities whenever necessary. In fact, they usually treat patients in more than one hospital. As such, they do not receive a salary from the hospital. Instead, they collect *fees* from their patients for their services.

A *medical director*, or *chief of staff*, oversees the staff of physicians. He or she is usually appointed by the hospital board. Sometimes the physicians recommend a member of the medical staff, and the board approves or disapproves. The medical director is responsible to the hospital board, and not to the hospital administrator. These two employees, however, must obviously work together to enable the hospital to deliver adequate and efficient health care.

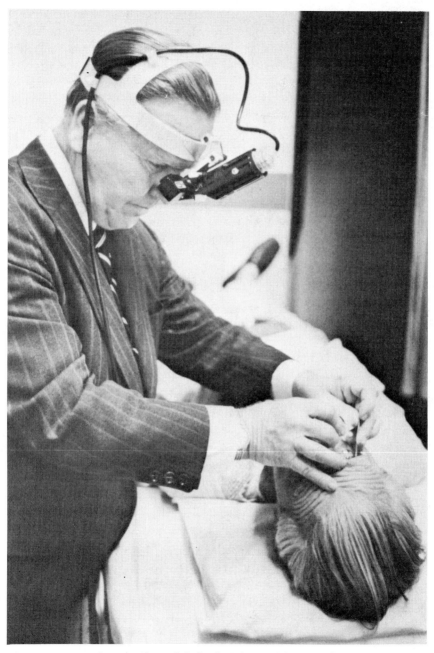

A physician (an ophthalmologist) examining a patient.
(Courtesy Manhattan Eye, Ear and Throat Hospital)

In order to maintain high medical standards at a hospital, a *medical advisory board* meets regularly to advise the board of directors on medical policies. This board, also known as the *joint conference committee*, consists of the medical director, the hospital administrator, and a selected number of physicians who serve as the heads of various medical departments. The medical staff has several internal committees as well. They constantly review medical practices and the performance of the physicians. Any physician who fails to meet the hospital's medical standards is no longer allowed to use the hospital's facilities.

The most serious complaint that can be raised against a physician is the accusation of *malpractice*. A physician who practices medicine without a license, or one who leaves a surgical tool in a patient after an operation, for example, can be charged with malpractice. If it can be shown that the doctor was simply careless, the charge can be reduced to *negligence*. If the patient proves his charge in a court of law, the patient usually is awarded a large sum of money in compensation. As a result, hospitals and doctors protect themselves with malpractice insurance. It is a very costly but essential form of insurance.

A hospital cannot rely entirely on its consulting doctors for its medical services. It needs a permanent medical staff as well to provide continuous health care. Medical students, known as *interns* and *residents*, fill this role. Both interns and residents have successfully completed their academic studies. They have not yet been licensed, however, to practice medicine. A medical student must complete at least a year of internship at an accredited hospital before he can be licensed in most places in the United States. Most student interns rotate throughout the various medical departments to familiarize themselves with all aspects of the medical profession.

If a student chooses to specialize in one area of medicine, he becomes a resident physician in the hospital following his internship. For several years, he works in the specialty of his choice. When he has gotten enough experience, he can be licensed in that specialty.

The patient who is admitted to a hospital is viewed by the medical staff as a medical *case* with a problem to be solved. A doctor must then examine the patient in order to *diagnose* or determine what is wrong with him. Once a *diagnosis* has been made, the physician must then prescribe some form of *treatment* to cure the patient. This treatment may simply be medical, involving the use of medication. It

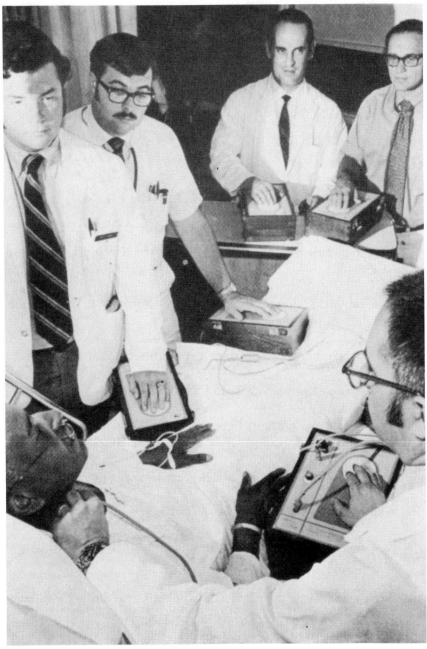

Residents attending a lecture at a patient's bedside. Each resident has his hand on a palpator, which enables a doctor to feel a human pulse by remote control.
(Courtesy Georgetown University Medical Center)

may also be surgical, necessitating an operation. Different kinds of therapy may also be involved. A good hospital can provide treatment in one of its many medical departments for whatever problem the patient has. The quality of the treatment largely reflects the quality of the medical staff working at the hospital.

Discussion

1. Which members of the hospital staff are the most essential to its purpose? Why?

2. What qualities must one have in order to become a successful doctor?

3. What is the minimum amount of schooling that a person must complete to become a doctor?

4. Does it take longer to become a specialist?

5. How are most physicians paid for their services?

6. What is the relationship between the medical director and the hospital administrator?

7. Explain how the medical staff in a hospital is organized.

8. What does the medical advisory board do?

9. How does a hospital control the standards of the medical care it offers?

10. What happens to a physician who fails to meet these standards?

11. Give an example of malpractice. How is negligence different?

12. How do doctors protect themselves against a malpractice suit?

13. Since most physicians are not employees of the hospital, who makes up the permanent medical staff of the hospital?

14. Explain the licensing procedure in the United States.

15. What must a doctor do before he can treat a patient?

Review

A. Describe some of the rewards and drawbacks of the medical profession. Are you a doctor (or studying to become one)? If so, why did you choose a career in medicine?

B. Divide up your class and assume the different roles on the medical advisory board. Have different people play the roles of the hospital administrator, the medical director, and the physicians serving as heads of the medical departments. One of the surgeons in your hospital has been threatened with a charge of malpractice. You as a board must decide whether to retain him on your staff, supporting him in his case, or to release him and defend the patient. The student playing the role of the head of surgery will present the case.

C. Are the following statements true or false? Explain your answers.

1. Being a doctor requires a great deal of dedication and a willingness to accept responsibility.

2. *Physician* is another name for a doctor of medicine.

3. Most physicians are paid by the hospital where they practice.

4. The medical staff in a hospital is supervised by the hospital administrator.

5. The joint conference committee advises the hospital board on medical policies.

6. A physician who practices without a license can be accused of malpractice.

7. Hospitals usually protect physicians against malpractice suits.

8. An intern has completed his medical degree but is not yet licensed to practice.

9. A doctor must spend several years as a resident physician in an approved hospital before becoming a licensed specialist.

10. A doctor must examine a patient completely before he knows what treatment to prescribe.

UNIT FIVE
THE NURSING STAFF

Special Terms

Nurse: Person trained to perform a variety of functions associated with the care of sick persons. The term is a broad one. It covers a wide range of positions that involve training in various specialties. Men who become nurses are called male nurses.

Director of Nursing: Nurse responsible for the nursing staff in a hospital.

Registered Professional Nurse: Nurse who has completed a two- to four-year course at an approved nursing school and has been licensed to practice after passing an official examination. Qualified to assume the most difficult nursing duties, he or she may also be referred to as either a *professional nurse* or an R.N.

Licensed Practical Nurse: Nurse who has completed a one-year course in nursing but cannot assume the same responsibilities as an R.N. He or she is known as an L.P.N.

Nurse's Aide: Person without a formal nursing degree who assists the nursing staff.

Orderly: Assists with various routine nursing duties. Orderlies usually perform the more physically difficult tasks, such as lifting and moving patients. They are usually male.

Blood Transfusion: Injection of bottled human blood into a patient. Transfusions are necessary when a patient has lost a substantial amount of blood.

I.V.: Abbreviation for *intravenous*. When a fluid is administered to a patient by means of a small tube or *catheter* directly into a vein, it is called an I.V.

Vital Signs: The indications of life in a patient. The *blood pressure*, the *pulse* or *heartbeat*, and the *temperature* must be checked regularly.

To Prep: To prepare a patient, as for an operation. This may include shaving hair, washing a body area, and so on.

Dressing: Another name for a bandage that usually covers the sutures or stitches after a surgical procedure.

Shift: Period of duty, usually eight hours long. Since nursing services must be provided continuously, each day is divided into three shifts.

On Duty: Term used to refer to the time when an employee is at work. The opposite is *off duty*.

Ward: A room with many beds. It can also mean a general area or wing of the hospital. Patients are hospitalized with other patients who have similar conditions. Hence, there is a maternity ward, a communicable disease ward, and so on.

Nurse's Station: A central area on the floor or ward where nurses are based.

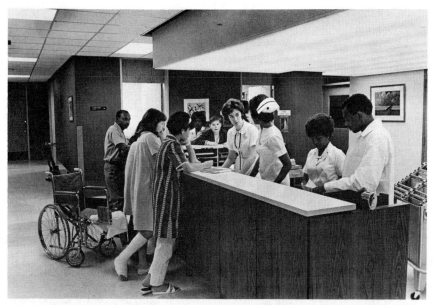

A typical nurse's station. (Courtesy Montefiore Hospital and Medical Center)

Intensive Care: Nursing care provided to the seriously ill patient during which constant attention is paid to the patient's condition.

Vocabulary Practice

1. What does a *nurse* do?

2. Do all nurses have the same training?

3. What is another name for a *professional nurse*?

4. What does *L.P.N.* stand for?

5. What is the difference between an R.N. and an L.P.N.?

6. Is it more difficult to become a nurse or a doctor?

7. What is a *nurse's aide*?

8. Who might be called to move a patient to the operating room?

9. When might a patient need a *blood transfusion*?

10. What is the common abbreviation for *intravenous*? What does it mean to administer a fluid intravenously?

11. Why must a patient's *vital signs* be checked regularly? Give an example of a vital sign.

12. When a nurse *preps* a patient, what may be involved?

13. What is another name for a surgical bandage?

14. How long is a nursing *shift* in most cases?

15. What is the opposite of *off duty*?

16. What is the *nurse's station?*

17. Why do you think patients are usually hospitalized in a *ward* with patients that have similar problems?

18. What is meant by *intensive care?*

The Nursing Staff

The physicians in a hospital form the core of the medical staff. But they could not provide effective medical care to their patients without the help of numerous other medical employees. From the viewpoint of the patients, the nursing staff is particularly important. Nurses are usually in close contact with patients as long as they are in the hospital.

A nurse does not study for as many years as a doctor. However, each must be equally dedicated. Caring for sick persons requires a

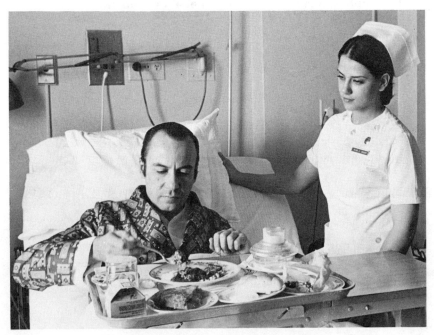

A nurse adjusting the pillows of a patient.
(Courtesy The New York Hospital—Cornell Medical Center)

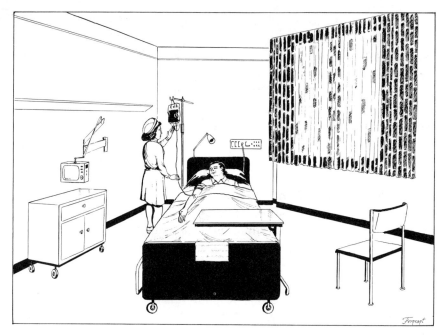

A nurse administering a transfusion to a patient.

great deal of patience and concern. Most nurses work long days, and they often must work at odd hours or during the night.

The nursing staff in a hospital is usually quite large and diverse. Nursing services, after all, must be provided on a 24-hour basis. There are professional nurses, practical nurses, nurse's aides, and orderlies. The general term *nurse* refers to a person trained to offer bedside care to sick persons.

To serve as a *director of nursing* in a hospital, one must be trained as a *registered professional nurse,* otherwise known as an *R.N.* To become a registered nurse, one must complete a two- to four-year program in an accredited nursing school. An R.N. assumes responsibility for a patient's needs, depending on the instructions of the attending physician. This kind of nurse also regularly administers medicine, assists with *blood transfusions,* and administers *I.V.'s.*

A *licensed practical nurse,* or *L.P.N.,* is allowed to practice after successfully completing a one-year program. The L.P.N. may make routine checks of a patient's *vital signs,* change a patient's surgical *dressings,* or *prep* a patient for surgery.

Other employees who come under the jurisdiction of the director of nursing are *aides* and *orderlies*. They perform routine functions to assist the R.N.'s and the L.P.N.'s. These may include feeding a patient or helping a patient get dressed.

Under the supervision of the head nurse, the nursing staff in a hospital *ward* must attend to patients' needs. This responsibility continues around the clock, and so nurses must work in shifts. A *shift* is a period of duty, usually eight hours in length. The nurses on the ward rotate their shifts. Some take turns working night duty; others work odd shifts. All of them work out of a central area on the ward called the *nurse's station.*

A nurse must always be alert. She can never afford to be careless. This is true in all nursing situations, but it is especially true in the *intensive care* unit. Patients under intensive care are critically ill, and they must be monitored at all times. The nurses who do intensive care duty have one of the most demanding jobs in the hospital.

Serving as a nurse on a hospital nursing staff can be a very rewarding job. But it is not an easy one. Not every person is suited to become a nurse. Only very dedicated people have chosen nursing as a profession.

Discussion

1. Do patients have a lot of contact with the nursing staff?

2. Does a nurse need the same training that a doctor needs?

3. Name some of the various types of nurses who make up the nursing staff in a hospital.

4. Which nurse has more training, a registered nurse or a licensed practical nurse?

5. When might a nurse have to give an I.V. to a patient?

6. What will a nurse be likely to do if she notices that a patient's vital signs are weakening?

7. Why does a nurse have to work at night from time to time?

8. What kind of patient might need to be confined to the intensive care unit?

Review

A. Name as many duties as you can think of that might be performed by a nurse for a patient. Which member of the nursing staff would perform each one?

B. Are you a nurse? If not, do you know anyone who is? How would you advise someone who asked you about the rewards and problems of nursing?

C. Match the following terms in the left column with the correct definition in the right column. Only one definition is appropriate for each term.

____ Shift	1. Injection of bottled human blood.
____ On Duty	2. Nurse with one year of training.
____ R.N.	3. Heartbeat, temperature, and blood pressure.
____ Orderly	4. Male attendant.
____ Ward	5. Eight-hour period of duty.
____ Vital Signs	6. At work.
____ I.V.	7. Bandage.
____ L.P.N.	8. Trained professional nurse.
____ Transfusion	9. Administering fluid by a catheter.
____ Dressing	10. Floor, wing, or large patient area.

UNIT SIX
MAJOR MEDICAL DEPARTMENTS

Special Terms

Medical Department: A division of medical services in the hospital that offers diagnosis and treatment in one area. Examples of medical departments include surgery, neurology, and pediatrics. These divisions may also be referred to as *clinical departments*. Each department is run by a senior physician known as the *head of the department*.

Surgery: The medical department responsible for performing operations on patients. During an *operation*, a medical problem is corrected with the use of surgical tools. Two common tools include the *scalpel*, which is a small knife, and the *forceps*, which is a set of tongs. A physician qualified to perform operations is known as a *surgeon*.

Exploratory Surgery: Surgery that is performed to help confirm a diagnosis. It usually is not intended to cure the patient.

Anesthesia: General or local insensibility to pain induced by certain drugs or gases called *anesthetics*. They are usually administered by a trained *anesthesiologist*, who is a doctor, or an *anesthetist*, who usually is not.

Patient Monitoring: The use of electronic devices to keep constant watch over a patient's vital signs.

Sterilization: The process of destroying disease-producing organisms, usually through the use of heat. Items that have been sterilized are said to be *sterile*.

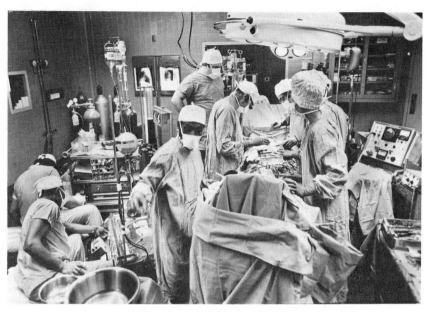

A typical operating room during an operation.
(Courtesy The New York Hospital—Cornell Medical Center)

Obstetrics: A medical term relating to the delivery of babies. A physician specializing in this area of medicine is an *obstetrician.*

Operating Room: A special room in a hospital equipped for operations.

Gynecology: The science of the female reproductive system. A *gynecologist* can usually deliver babies, as well as the obstetrician.

Labor: The series of contractions of the uterus prior to the birth of an infant.

Recovery Room: The room in which a patient recovers from an operation or recovers from the delivery of an infant.

Nursery: The place in which newborn babies are cared for after their delivery. Most hospitals have regular nurseries and *premature* nurseries for babies who are born before the end of the normal nine-month gestation period.

Maternity Floor: The part of the hospital where mothers give birth to babies and are cared for afterward. Most women spend from a few days to a week here. This area may also be referred to as a *ward* or a *wing.*

Cesarean Section: A method of delivering a child that involves cutting into the uterus. The name comes from the supposed fact that Julius Caesar was delivered this way.

Rooming-in: A new practice that allows newborn infants to spend much of their time in their mothers' rooms.

Pediatrician: A doctor who specializes in the care of children from the time they are born until they are teenagers. Most general hospitals have a separate *pediatrics* department.

General Medicine: A term covering a broad range of medical services offered by a hospital. Patients in this department are cured by medicine or another form of therapy.

Internist: A doctor who specializes in general, internal problems that can be cured by medication.

Dermatologist: A specialist in skin problems. *Dermatology* is the study and treatment of skin problems.

Communicable Diseases: Diseases that are infectious or can spread from one patient to another. Included in this category are measles, smallpox, poliomyelitis, meningitis, and so on.

Vocabulary Practice

1. Name several *medical departments* in a hospital.

2. What does a *surgeon* do?

3. What are *scalpels* and *forceps*?

4. How can *exploratory surgery* help with a diagnosis of a patient's problems?

5. Where do operations take place?

6. What is the purpose of an *anesthetic*? Who administers it?

7. Explain *patient monitoring*.

8. Why must all tools used in an operation be *sterilized*?

9. What physician specializes in the delivery of babies?

10. Can a *gynecologist* also deliver babies? What is his specialty?

11. What is *labor*?

12. What wing in the hospital takes care of pregnant women before and after the delivery of their babies?

13. What is the *recovery room*?

14. How does a *Cesarean section* differ from normal childbirth?

15. Where are newborn infants cared for?

16. What is *rooming-in*?

17. What specialist assumes responsibility for a child once it is born?

18. How does *general medicine* differ from *surgery*?

19. What does an *internist* do? A *dermatologist*?

20. Name some *communicable diseases.*

Major Medical Departments

No hospital is able to deal with all the medical problems that mankind is susceptible to. The community hospital can usually handle most problems, as long as they are not extremely specialized or complicated. Other hospitals provide care to only one kind of patient—the mentally ill, for example, or perhaps maternity cases. The size of the hospital often reflects the variety of care it can offer.

Most community hospitals, no matter how small, have at least the following major *medical departments:* surgery, obstetrics and gynecology, pediatrics, and general medicine. Each of these departments is run by a senior physician called the *department head.* The department heads are supervised by the hospital's medical director.

The medical department that is probably the best known is *surgery,* perhaps because of its dramatic nature. The doctors in this division perform operations on patients when they are needed. Almost half of all patients admitted to a hospital have operations. Many of the terms frequently heard in conversations, such as *scalpel* or *forceps*, are related to this area of specialization.

A physician whose specialty is surgery is known as a *surgeon*. Usually, a patient is referred to a surgeon once it has been determined that he may need an operation. Sometimes the surgeon operates

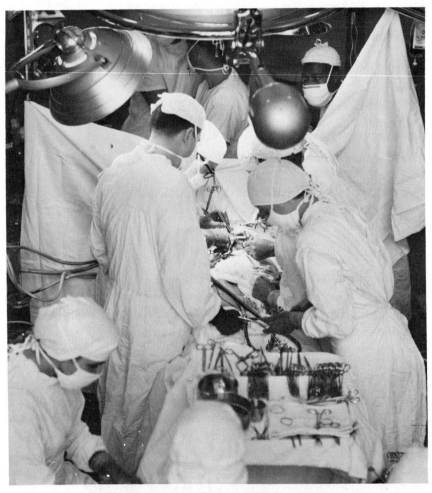

Surgeons performing open heart surgery.
(Courtesy The New York Hospital—Cornell Medical Center)

immediately to cure the patient. He or she may also wish to confirm the tentative diagnosis first with *exploratory surgery.*

Within the field of surgery, there are many specialties. A surgeon who specializes in fixing broken bones, for example, is called an *orthopedic* surgeon. One who operates on nervous disorders is a *neurosurgeon.* A surgeon who treats just chest and lung problems is a *thoracic* surgeon. And a surgeon whose specialty is repairing injured or malformed organs or tissues is a *plastic* surgeon.

The surgeons in a hospital make the greatest use of the *operating room.* An operating room must be equipped with a variety of expensive equipment and tools. Because of constant technical advances, many operating suites quickly become obsolete.

One of the most important aspects of surgery involves the *anesthesiologist* or *anesthetist.* In the early days of medical care, operations were performed without the benefit of an *anesthetic.* Patients thus suffered considerable pain. Today the administration of *anesthesia* has become so important, it is now recognized as a medical specialty.

Many operating rooms have traditionally been arranged with viewing galleries. They allow medical and nursing students to observe and learn from operations. As a result, they have been known as *operating theaters.* They are being used less frequently, however, due to the widespread use of closed circuit television.

The technique of *patient monitoring* has become very popular in operating rooms and other areas of the hospital. A patient's vital signs are constantly observed through the use of electronic devices attached to the patient. In this way, operating room attendants can alert surgeons immediately to changes in the patient's condition. Patient monitoring is a significant aid in improving a patient's chances of recovery.

The danger of infection during an operation is great. As a result, everything in the operating room must be *sterilized.* In addition, doctors, nurses, and attendants in the operating room must wear sterile gowns and special masks on their faces. These precautions add to the atmosphere of drama that surrounds the hospital's surgical department.

Another familiar medical department is the one that handles obstetrical and gynecological cases. *Obstetrics* is the medical term related to the delivery of babies. *Gynecology* is the science of the female reproductive system. *Obstetricians* and *gynecologists* are often skilled in both specialties.

Most women visit their "ob/gyn specialist" on a regular basis in his or her office. They are asked to use a hospital only if they need an operation or if they are ready to give birth to a child. A pregnant woman is admitted to a hospital once she has begun *labor*. She spends most of her time in a labor room and is moved to the *delivery room* only when the baby is ready to be born. The mother recovers for a short time after the delivery in a *recovery room*. The baby is taken immediately to a *nursery*.

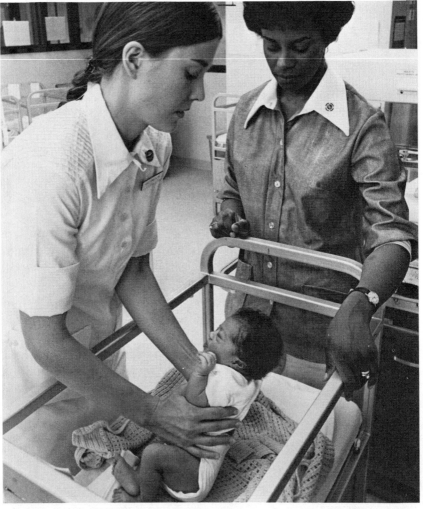

A nursery on a maternity floor. (Courtesy Georgetown University Medical Center)

A new mother spends between three days and a week on the *maternity floor* before she goes home. If she had a normal delivery, she only needs a few days. If a *Cesarean section* was necessary, she needs the full week. If the child was delivered prematurely, it has to be given special care in the premature nursery until strong enough to go home.

More and more hospitals are encouraging fathers to be present during labor and delivery. Hospitals are also making *rooming-in* facilities available for newborns. These programs help to make the hospital experience as comfortable as and similar to the home environment as possible.

The obstetrician or gynecologist is responsible for both the mother and the child during labor and delivery. However, once the baby is born, the *pediatrician* assumes responsibility for the care of the child. A pediatrician is a doctor who cares for children from the time they are born until they are teenagers. Parents usually bring their children to visit their pediatrician on a regular basis. Only very sick or injured children are admitted to the pediatrics department of the hospital. Most hospitals have special children's wards. The atmos-

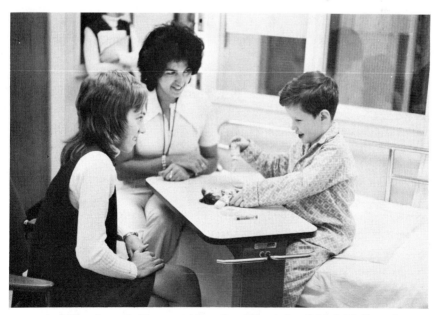

A children's ward. (Courtesy Montefiore Hospital and Medical Center)

phere there is made as pleasant as possible to encourage recovery. Arrangements often are made for parents to spend the night with their child.

The term *general medicine* is a broad one that covers some of the more ordinary medical services offered by a hospital. This last major medical department handles cases that can be treated medically, not surgically. Patients who have intestinal problems that can be treated with medication, for example, are the concern of this department. They are seen by the *internist.* Those with skin problems visit the *dermatologist.* Eye-ear-nose-and-throat specialists belong to the general medical staff. Patients suffering from allergies, venereal disease, glandular problems, and countless other ailments are treated here. In smaller hospitals, the department of general medicine handles a wide variety of patients. In larger hospitals, many of the services offered by this department are handled by independent, specialized departments.

Discussion

1. Can any hospital treat all the problems that people are susceptible to?

2. What medical departments do almost all community hospitals have?

3. Why is surgery one of the best known hospital departments?

4. Almost half of all patients admitted to a hospital have an operation performed. What is meant by the term *operation?*

5. When will a surgeon use exploratory surgery?

6. Are all surgeons able to handle all surgical problems? What are some subspecialties within surgery?

7. What benefit does a patient derive from an anesthetic?

8. Why have operating rooms often been called *operating theaters?*

9. One of the most recent technological advances in health care has been the development of patient monitoring. Why is it especially useful?

10. Most babies are born in hospitals in the United States. What medical department handles their delivery?

11. What does *rooming-in* mean? Why have many hospitals recently made facilities available for rooming-in, as well as encouraged fathers to be present at the birth?

12. What medical specialist assumes responsibility for a baby after its birth?

13. What is the major difference between the forms of treatment offered by the divisions of surgery and general medicine?

14. Does a patient usually receive more specialized care in a small hospital or a large one?

Review

A. Choose the appropriate answer or answers for each of the following. More than one choice may be correct.

    1. A _____ hospital can usually treat most patients.
      a) long-term care
      b) maternity
      c) community

    2. Which of the following departments are found in most community hospitals?
      a) obstetrics and gynecology
      b) ophthalmology
      c) surgery
      d) neurology
      e) pediatrics
      f) general medicine

g) psychiatry
h) nuclear medicine

3. Which of the following terms refer to a surgical specialty?
   a) orthopedic
   b) Cesarean
   c) dermatological
   d) plastic

4. Which of the following is likely to be found in an operating room?
   a) scalpel
   b) anesthesia
   c) nursery
   d) measles

5. Communicable diseases such as _____ often require hospitalization.
   a) pregnancy
   b) polio
   c) smallpox
   d) allergy

6. Which of the following disorders are treated by the department of general medicine?
   a) amputation
   b) gland problem
   c) skin problem
   d) pregnancy

7. Which terms refer to obstetrics and gynecology?
   a) labor
   b) internist
   c) Cesarean
   d) maternity

B. An operation is a very dramatic event. Have you ever seen one? Describe what you saw. What impressed you the most? Have you ever had an operation?

C. You are an internist. Another member of your class is a patient. He or she comes to you complaining of a pain in the stomach. Ask as many questions as you can to determine what is really wrong. Once you have a tentative diagnosis, suggest a possible treatment. If you cannot diagnose the problem, suggest an appropriate specialist for your patient to consult.

UNIT SEVEN
SPECIALIZED MEDICAL SERVICES

Special Terms

Cardiology: Medical specialty focusing on heart problems. A physician who practices this specialty is a *cardiologist.*

Electrocardiograph: Machine that records heart movements through electronic impulses. It is used in the diagnosis of heart problems. An *electrocardiogram* is recorded on paper as the result of the electrocardiograph. An *electrocardiograph technician* helps with the use of this *ECG* or *EKG* machine, as it is often called.

Endocrinologist: Specialist in *endocrinology,* the study of glandular problems.

Gastroenterologist: Specialist in *gastroenterology,* the study of diseases of the digestive organs.

Ophthalmologist: Specialist in *ophthalmology,* which deals with the structure, function, and diseases of the eye.

Dentist: A doctor who treats the teeth and tissues of the mouth. He is helped in his work by a *dental hygienist.* The medical specialty is *dentistry.*

Physical Medicine: Department specializing in rehabilitative services. *Physical therapy* utilizes heat, massage, and exercise to rehabilitate muscles, nerves, and bones. *Occupational therapy* helps to rehabilitate patients by keeping them busy with crafts.

Psychiatry: Division of medicine dedicated to the treatment of mental disorders. A specialist is a *psychiatrist.*

Electroencephalograph: Machine that records brain waves through electronic impulses. It produces a tracing on paper called an

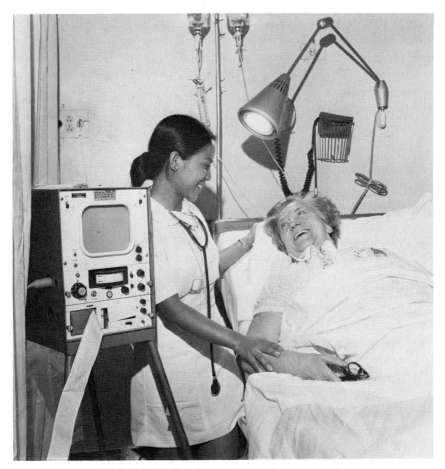

A nurse at a patient's bedside. Note the *electrocardiograph* on the left.
(Courtesy The New York Hospital—Cornell Medical Center)

electroencephalogram. The *EEG*, as it is often called, can help the
psychiatrist diagnose brain diseases.

Geriatrics: Medical specialty dealing with the diseases of aging. A
specialist in this area is a *geriatrician.*

Neurology: Branch of medicine dealing with the nervous system. The
neurologist specializes in this branch of medicine.

Urology: Branch of medicine dealing with the bladder and urinary
system. The doctor who specializes in this branch is called a
urologist.

Pulmonary Medicine: Study of lung ailments.

Renal Medicine: Study of kidney diseases.

Epidemiology: Study of the prevention and control of epidemic diseases. The doctor specializing in this kind of study is an *epidemiologist.*

Vocabulary Practice

1. What medical problems does a *cardiologist* treat?

2. What machine can a cardiologist use to help him with his diagnoses? What does this machine produce on paper?

3. What is the name for a specialist in the study of glandular diseases? A specialist in the study of digestive problems?

4. Define *endocrinology, gastroenterology,* and *ophthalmology.*

5. Who helps a *dentist* in his work?

6. Name two kinds of therapy used to rehabilitate patients. What techniques are used with each?

7. What is wrong with a patient treated by a *psychiatrist?*

8. What is an *EEG?* Whom does it help?

9. Define *geriatrics.*

10. Name and define some other specialized medical services that might be found in a hospital.

Specialized Medical Services

As a hospital expands, it usually offers additional specialized medical services. Many of the services once offered by the department of general medicine become medical departments of their own. A patient with a heart condition in a small community hospital is treated by the general medical staff. In a larger and more sophisticated hospital, he is probably cared for by the *cardiologist*, a heart specialist. The cardiologist is a member of the *cardiology department*, which is separate from the department of medicine.

When a hospital expands its services, the need for better-trained personnel and more sophisticated equipment increases. The cardiologist, for instance, makes use of a machine known as an *electrocardiograph*. This machine records heart actions through electronic impulses. An *electrocardiograph technician* attaches small electrodes to the patient's legs, arms, and chest. As the heart beats, the movements are recorded on paper as waves. This is known as an *electrocardiogram*. This *ECG* or *EKG*, as it is often called, can help a cardiologist make a diagnosis. In a smaller hospital, the patient with a heart condition would probably not have the benefit of this technique.

Other elements within the department of general medicine may become separate services. A hospital may have a department of *endocrinology* to treat glandular disorders. A *gastroenterologist* handles patients with intestinal or digestive problems. An *ophthalmologist* treats eye diseases, and a *dermatologist* sees patients complaining of skin problems. There may be many more. The variety of specialized services depends on the size of the hospital.

A department of *dentistry* is not always found in hospitals. The reason for this is the fact that most people prefer to visit their *dentist* in his private office. The dentist of course treats oral health problems. With the assistance of a *dental hygienist*, he or she locates and fills cavities, extracts teeth, straightens crooked teeth, treats gum and mouth diseases, and provides artificial or false teeth. Modern dentists emphasize treatment *and* prevention of disorders of the mouth.

Rehabilitative services are available to any patient who is occupying a bed in a hospital. Patients who live at home use the hospital's facilities regularly as well. Several kinds of service are offered by the department of physical medicine: *physical therapy, occupational therapy, speech therapy, music therapy,* and so on. All therapists try to help patients regain their health as quickly as possible. They use a variety of techniques.

A physical therapist works to rehabilitate patients whose injuries or diseases affect the normal functioning of muscles, joints, nerves, or bones. The treatment itself often involves the use of exercise, massage,

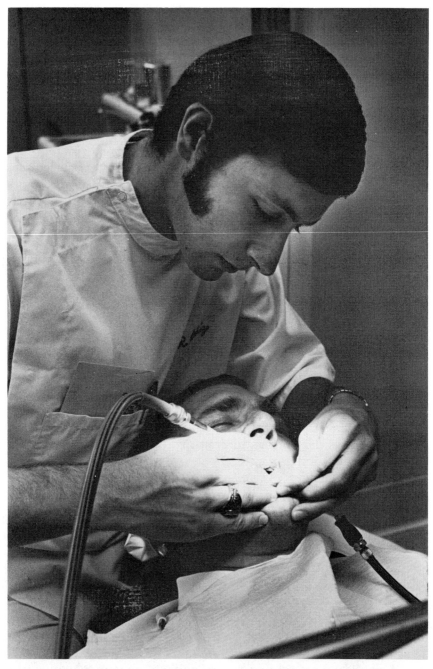

A dentist. (Courtesy Georgetown University Medical Center)

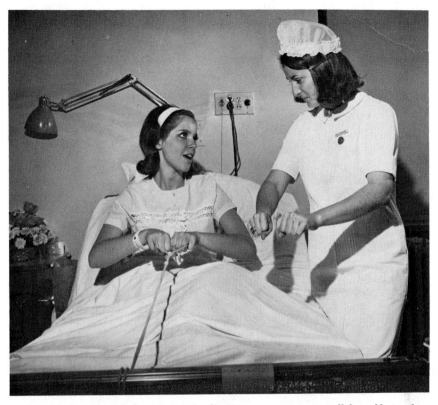

A physical therapist teaching a patient how to use a rope to pull herself up after surgery. (Courtesy The New York Hospital—Cornell Medical Center)

heat, and cold. A great deal of patience is required by this kind of work. However, the rewards of watching and participating in a patient's recovery are highly satisfying. Physical therapists are well trained in their field, but they are not physicians. As a result, they always work closely with their patient's physician.

A hospital patient who is kept busy and free from worry will recover from an ailment more easily than a patient who is unoccupied. This is the basis of occupational therapy. Occupational therapists involve patients in different kinds of activities, usually crafts like weaving, woodworking, or needlework.

Some general hospitals have *psychiatric departments,* which treat patients who have mental disorders. Some psychiatric patients have chronic emotional problems, and they require long-term care. These

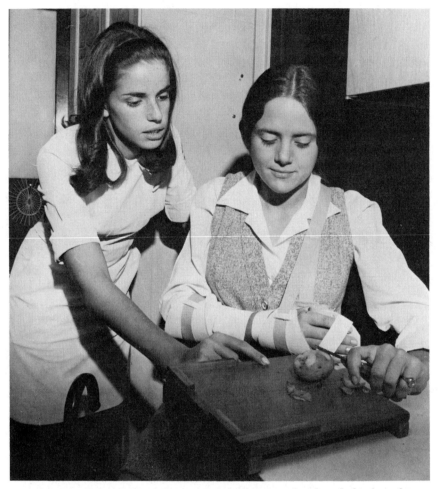

An occupational therapist teaching a patient to use one hand to do kitchen chores.
(Courtesy The New York Hospital—Cornell Medical Center)

kinds of patients are usually referred to hospitals that specialize in mental health care.

Trained *psychiatrists* treat patients with a variety of techniques. Today, utilizing the *electroencephalograph* can help the psychiatrist diagnose various brain diseases such as epilepsy, brain tumors, or strokes. This machine records brain waves through the use of small electrodes that are attached to the patient's scalp. The resultant tracings create the *electroencephalogram,* or *EEG.* Special technicians generally help the psychiatrist use the machine.

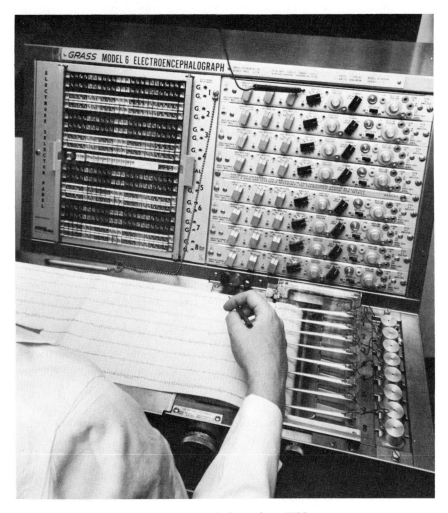

An electroencephalograph or EEG.
(Courtesy Montefiore Hospital and Medical Center)

Thanks primarily to medical science, people live longer than they used to. As a result, a medical specialty called *geriatrics* is attracting a great deal of attention. This relatively new branch of medicine focuses on the health problems of the elderly. Specialists called *geriatricians* are being trained, and increasing attention is being paid to the needs of the aged in hospitals.

The specialties referred to here are only a few of the many specialized medical services that might be found in a hospital. Others include *neurology, urology, pulmonary medicine, renal medicine, epidemiology,* and so on. The services offered by any particular hospital depend on many factors: its size, the community it serves, its financial resources, the availability of trained specialists, and the interests of its board of directors.

Discussion

1. What usually happens to the services offered by the department of general medicine as a hospital grows in size?

2. If you were a patient with a heart problem in a small community hospital, which department would care for you? Would this be true in a large hospital?

3. How does an electrocardiograph help a cardiologist with his diagnoses?

4. Name some other functions of the department of general medicine that may become specialized departments in a larger hospital.

5. Do most people have their dental problems cared for in a hospital or in a dentist's private office? Why?

6. Name some of the things a dentist will do in treating the mouth and teeth.

7. When is physical therapy used?

8. What kinds of treatment does a physical therapist employ?

9. Why do you think a physical therapist needs a great deal of patience?

10. What is the basis of occupational therapy?

11. Why are patients with chronic psychiatric problems sent to specialized hospitals?

12. Explain how an electroencephalograph works.

13. Why has a specialty called geriatrics been developed recently?

Review

A. Complete the following statements with appropriate words or expressions.

1. A patient with a mental disorder is treated by a
   _____.

2. An _____ is a tracing on paper of a patient's heart movements.

3. Modern dentists emphasize _____ as well as treatment of mouth disorders.

4. As a hospital grows in size, the number of specialized medical services _____.

5. A medical specialty focusing on the problems of the elderly is known as _____.

6. _____ therapy involves the use of crafts.

B. As a member of the hospital board, you have been asked to consider establishing a mental health wing in the hospital to handle psychiatric patients. You do not think this is a good idea. What are some of your reasons?

C. Try to think of other health problems, diseases, or physical ailments that you have heard of. Are there medical specialists to treat them? If so, name them.

UNIT EIGHT
ADDITIONAL SUPPORTING UNITS
AND SERVICES

Special Terms

Paramedical: Related to the medical profession in a supporting or supplementary manner. A paramedical technician has some training in his specialty, but not as much as a doctor. This kind of technician is often now called an *allied health professional.*

Anesthesiologist: Doctor trained in the administration of *anesthetics,* drugs or gases—such as ether—that produce *anesthesia* or insensitivity to pain.

Radiologist: Specialist in the use of *x rays.* These rays are given off by various radioactive substances. They are used to photograph bones and inner organs. All radiologists are physicians.

Nuclear Medicine: New medical specialty featuring the use of radioactive isotopes for diagnostic purposes. The isotope is injected into skin tissue, the bloodstream, or an organ. Its movement is followed by a device known as a *scanner.*

Laboratory: Area in the hospital responsible for analyzing samples of blood, urine, tissue, and so on. These samples are called *specimens.* The *lab* is run by a *pathologist,* a doctor who interprets and diagnoses diseases by examining samples of tissue, blood, and so on. The lab is staffed by *laboratory technicians.*

Urinalysis: Laboratory analysis of a urine specimen.

Microscope: A device used in laboratory analyses that magnifies what is too small for the eye to see.

Centrifuge: An apparatus that separates substances of different densities by rotating at high speeds. It is used in a hospital laboratory.

Autopsy: Examination of a body after death to determine the cause of death. The body is kept in the hospital *morgue* during the autopsy and until it is removed for burial.

Medical Audit: Professional evaluation of the quality of medical care offered to patients.

Basal Metabolism Rate: The speed at which a body at rest uses oxygen to consume the calories in food.

Blood Bank: Storage place for bottled human blood to be used in *transfusions*. The laboratory in a hospital is responsible for this blood.

Pharmacy: Area in a hospital where medication is prepared and dispensed by a trained *pharmacist*.

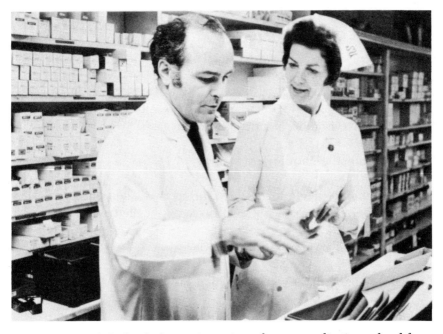

A pharmacist and the head of a nursing unit confer over medication ordered for a patient. (Courtesy Manhattan Eye, Ear and Throat Hospital)

Prescription: A written order for medication. A physician writes the prescription and a pharmacist fills it.

Oxygen Therapy: Administration of oxygen—to patients who are having trouble breathing—through the use of an *oxygen tent* or *mask*.

Renal Dialysis: Procedure used by patients who have lost the use of their kidneys. Their kidney function must be replaced two or three times a week by a renal dialysis machine.

Vocabulary Practice

1. Define *paramedical*. What are paramedical technicians now often called?

2. Are employees working in paramedical capacities likely to have medical degrees?

3. What is the name for a drug or a gas such as ether that causes *anesthesia*?

4. What is an *x ray* specialist called?

5. What is the name of a new medical specialty featuring the use of radioactive isotopes for diagnostic purposes?

6. Who runs the hospital *laboratory*?

7. Give another name for a blood, urine, or tissue sample. What is the laboratory analysis of a urine sample called?

8. What do *laboratory technicians* do?

9. Name and define two devices that are used in a laboratory.

10. When is an *autopsy* performed? Why?

11. Where is a body kept during an *autopsy*?

12. Define *medical audit*.

13. What does a *basal metabolism* machine measure?

14. Where is the bottled blood used in *transfusions* kept?

15. Who prepares and dispenses medication?

16. How does a physician communicate his needs to the pharmacist?

17. When is an *oxygen tent* or *mask* used?

18. What organs are not functioning properly if a patient must undergo *renal dialysis* treatments?

Additional Supporting Units and Services

A hospital cannot function without physicians and nurses to provide medical care. An extensive administrative and institutional staff is also necessary to run the hospital. But this is still not enough. Other staff members and facilities must be available to support the medical staff. The *anesthesiologist* or *anesthetist* prepares patients for surgery by making them insensitive to pain. The *radiologist* or *x-ray technician* takes x rays and interprets them. A staff of *laboratory technicians* analyzes *specimens* of blood, urine, and tissues taken from patients. A *pharmacist* prepares medication and dispenses it from the hospital *pharmacy*. Some of these services and others like them are called *paramedical* because they require *some* medical training. Those people who provide administrative and institutional services do not need medical training.

An anesthesiologist is trained in the administration of *anesthetics*, which are drugs or gases that render a patient insensitive to pain. There are two kinds of anesthesia. One is general, affecting the entire body; the other is local, temporarily deadening just the relevant area. Anesthetics are used most commonly in the operating room. Until recently, the surgeon used to administer the drug or gas himself. But the science of anesthesia is very complex, so an anesthesiologist or anesthetist is nearly always required today. An anesthetist is not a medical doctor, but he must be trained in his specialty and licensed before he can be hired. This is true of all of the paramedical technicians.

A hospital's department of radiology or x-ray department is

supervised by a radiologist. With the assistance of paramedical x-ray technicians, bones and inner organs of the human body are photographed. This technique is extremely helpful in diagnosis. The x ray can also be used therapeutically. However, x rays are extremely potent, and people must not be exposed to them too often or for too long. Everyone who works closely with them must take precautions to avoid overexposure.

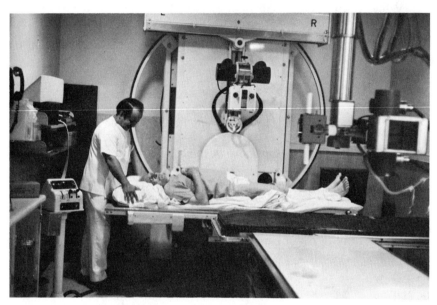

An x-ray technician preparing a patient for an x ray.
(Courtesy Montefiore Hospital and Medical Center)

A new specialty closely related to radiology is *nuclear medicine*. This involves a diagnostic technique during which a radioactive isotope is injected into the bloodstream, tissue, or organ that is being examined. Most new hospitals have independent departments of nuclear medicine, and many older hospitals are recognizing their usefulness.

The *laboratory* is the province of the *pathologist*, who is always a physician, and a staff of skilled paramedical laboratory technicians. Here, various specimens of blood, urine, and tissue are analyzed. Such valuable tools as the *microscope* and the *centrifuge* are utilized in the lab. The results of lab analysis provide physicians with valuable information that they can use as a guide in diagnosis and treatment. Medicine today requires more and more laboratory work. One of the

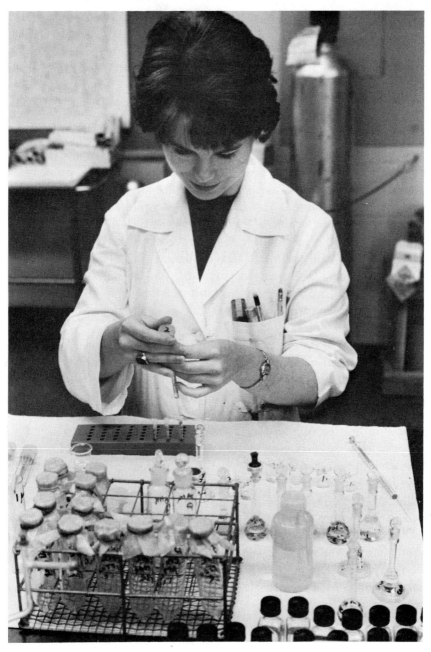

A lab technician. (Courtesy Montefiore Hospital and Medical Center)

great advantages of modern hospital care is the availability of this kind of service.

The pathologist who runs the lab is trained in the study of the cause of disease. Unlike many of the other doctors on the hospital staff, he may be employed by the hospital on a salary basis. The pathologist's duties are so important to the hospital that a hospital usually prefers him to be a permanent staff member.

In addition to running the laboratory, the pathologist is very involved in *medical audit* procedures. After a patient dies, for example, an *autopsy* may be performed to determine the exact cause of death. The body is transported to the morgue, where it is dissected and carefully examined. Tissue and blood samples are microscopically analyzed in the laboratory. The body is kept in the morgue until the autopsy is completed. Then it may be removed for burial.

Of course, the assumed cause of death is not always the same as the actual cause. Learning the true cause can be helpful to scientific research. Autopsies are also essential to the evaluation of the medical care offered by a hospital. They provide crucial evidence in malpractice cases too.

In most hospitals, the laboratory is also responsible for performing basal metabolism tests on patients. The *basal metabolism rate* indicates the patient's rate of oxygen use as he consumes the calories provided by food. This rate is tested while the patient is at rest. In addition, the laboratory usually maintains the *blood bank*—a supply of bottled human blood used in giving transfusions.

Another essential service is the *pharmacy*, where medication is prepared and dispensed for the hospital's patients. When a physician decides what medicine will benefit his patient, he writes an order called a *prescription*. It is then filled by the *pharmacist*. The medication often needs to be specially prepared.

Paramedical support units make the greatest use of technical equipment in the hospital, such as the *oxygen tent* and *mask*. Another of the pieces of equipment requiring special training is the *renal dialysis* machine. Patients who have lost the use of their kidneys must use this machine to remove waste materials from their bodies. Although some patients have installed the machines in their homes, most patients visit a hospital two or three times per week. Patients spend an average of four to six hours with the machine during each visit. A trained hospital staff is essential to this service.

Advances in medical science have greatly increased the quality of medical care available to hospital patients. Many of these advances,

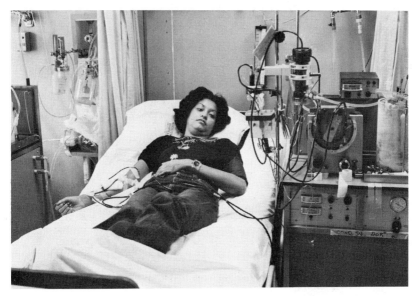

A patient undergoing renal dialysis.
(Courtesy Montefiore Hospital and Medical Center)

however, involve the use of special equipment and techniques. They also require specially trained personnel. The advantage of the modern hospital is that a wide range of these services and personnel are available to its patients. In fact, these facilities and the people who operate them have become so essential that most hospitals cannot function very effectively without them.

Discussion

1. Explain the difference between a paramedical and an administrative service.

2. What is the purpose of anesthetics?

3. What do you think are the dangers in administering anesthetics?

4. What does an x ray photograph?

5. Are x rays only used for diagnoses, or can they be used therapeutically as well?

6. Can a person be exposed to an unlimited number of x rays?

7. What new specialty utilizes radioactive isotopes? Explain how this specialty works.

8. How can the urinalyses, blood counts, and other tests performed by lab technicians be of help to a physician?

9. What does a pathologist do?

10. Why are autopsies performed?

11. Explain what is done during the autopsy.

12. What is the blood bank?

13. Who determines what medication a patient should be given, the pharmacist or the physician?

Review

A. Match the following terms in the left column with the correct definition in the right column. Only one definition is appropriate for each term.

____ Basal Metabolism	1. Device used in nuclear medicine.
____ Oxygen Tent	2. Study of the nature and cause of diseases.
____ Prescription	3. Device used to magnify small particles.
____ Radiologist	4. Technique used by kidney patients.
____ Specimen	5. Sample of fluid or tissue.
____ Pathology	6. Order for medication.
____ Morgue	7. Rate at which a body uses oxygen.

_____ Microscope

_____ Renal Dialysis

_____ Scanner

8. Used by patients suffering from lack of air.
9. Specialist in x-ray techniques.
10. Place where bodies are kept before burial.

B. Complete the following statements with an appropriate word or expression.

1. The analysis of urine performed by a laboratory technician is called _____.

2. Prior to surgery, an _____ administers a drug to a patient to render him insensitive to pain.

3. A centrifuge is used by a _____.

4. A picture taken of a patient's bones is called an _____.

5. An _____ is useful in conducting a medical audit.

6. A _____ technician has some training in the field of medicine, but not as much as a doctor.

7. The laboratory is run by a _____.

8. Bottled blood from the blood bank is used in the administration of _____.

9. X rays can be used for _____ as well as diagnoses.

C. A patient has just died in the hospital where you are working. Explain what procedures will be followed. Try to imagine all of the implications of this death. Could the responsible doctor be sued for malpractice? Should a medical audit be made to assure

the hospital board that medical practices are still of high quality?
Discuss the following in connection with this event:

1. the pathologist's role
2. an autopsy
3. malpractice
4. malpractice insurance
5. the medical review committee

UNIT NINE
OUTPATIENT AND EMERGENCY
SERVICES

Special Terms

Outpatient: A patient who uses the hospital's facilities but lives at home. An *inpatient* has access to the hospital's facilities also, but he or she stays in the hospital.

Extended Care Facilities: Hospital facilities where skilled nursing and related medical care services are continuously available to patients who do not require the complete diagnostic and treatment facilities of the hospital. These facilities are also known as *outpatient facilities.*

Ambulatory: Able to walk; not confined to bed. Patients who make use of outpatient or extended care services usually are ambulatory.

Self-care Patient: A patient who must continue regular treatments at the outpatient facilities but who does not need much assistance from the medical staff.

Progressive Hospital Care: The concept of treating a person only as much as is necessary. Patients remain inpatients until they no longer need the facilities of the hospital. Then they take advantage of the hospital's facilities on an outpatient basis.

Emergency Unit: Special facility in a hospital where ailments are treated 24 hours a day, 7 days a week.

Ambulance: An auto that transports the sick or injured—usually at high speeds—to a hospital. An ambulance is allowed to violate traffic regulations in the interest of the health of the patient, using a siren to warn other vehicles of its approach. Most ambulances are equipped with immediate care equipment.

Vocabulary Practice

1. What is an *outpatient?* An *inpatient?*

2. Give another name for *outpatient facilities.*

3. What does it mean to be *ambulatory?*

4. Are most patients who use outpatient services ambulatory?

5. What is a *self-care patient?*

6. Explain the concept of *progressive hospital care.*

7. What is the purpose of the *emergency unit?*

8. What is an *ambulance?* How does it warn other vehicles of its approach?

Outpatient and Emergency Services

Health care is improving everywhere. Additional kinds of facilities, such as clinics, are being built every day. Still, the hospital remains the most prominent health care agency. Small clinics usually cannot afford to maintain all the sophisticated equipment now available for treatment.

Hospitals do not have unlimited bed space for patients. In fact, many hospitals are unable to accommodate all of their patients. As a result, more and more hospitals are developing *outpatient* or *extended care facilities.* Rather than enter as an *inpatient,* the patient visits the hospital only if further diagnosis or treatment is necessary. In this way, patients who do not require the regular supervision of the hospital staff can still benefit from the facilities available at the hospital. In addition, beds can be reserved for the acutely ill. Patients may even save as much as half of the money they would normally have to pay for inpatient treatment.

Patients who use outpatient services are usually *ambulatory,* or able to walk. Among them are persons who have just completed a

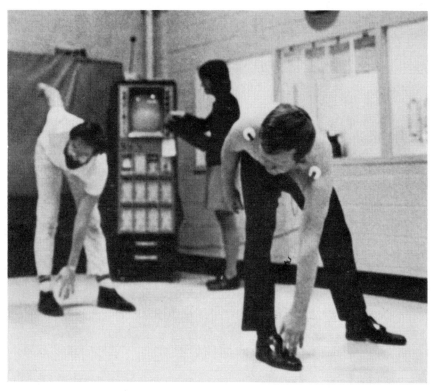

Ambulatory, self-care patients exercising under the supervision of a nurse at an outpatient facility. (Courtesy Montefiore Hospital and Medical Center)

hospital stay during the acute phase of an illness and who need some follow-up treatment. Patients hospitalized for a stroke or a heart attack fall into this category.

The elderly also are making greater use of various forms of extended care facilities. Medical advances enable people to live longer, but they often have chronic health problems—such as high blood pressure or rheumatism—that require constant supervision but not hospitalization. In the United States, Medicare has made it possible for the elderly to take advantage of these health facilities.

Facilities for *self-care patients* are also included in the outpatient centers. Included are the diabetic learning to give himself insulin; the post-coronary patient trying to adjust to a new pace of life; and the patient requiring regular x-ray therapy. Each kind of patient is encouraged to live as normal a life as possible, using the hospital's facilities only when necessary. This concept is known as *progressive hospital care.*

Outpatient services are utilized in other ways. The rehabilitation facilities of the physical medicine department—including physical, occupational, and speech therapy—are often used on an outpatient basis. Psychiatric day care is an outpatient service. Many persons who have psychiatric problems are not sick enough to be confined in a mental health unit, but they do require the support and counsel of trained psychiatric personnel. Where a hospital has a psychiatric outpatient service, these individuals can visit on a regular basis, receiving the appropriate amount of care. The cost is minimal and, more importantly, the patients are not completely removed from their normal environment. Dental care, eye-ear-nose-and-throat care, and so on are also available as outpatient services.

The *emergency units* in hospitals are becoming very popular. These facilities have always been well used for the critically ill or injured. Now, however, people are using them more and more as a convenient place to get treatment for noncritical conditions. The

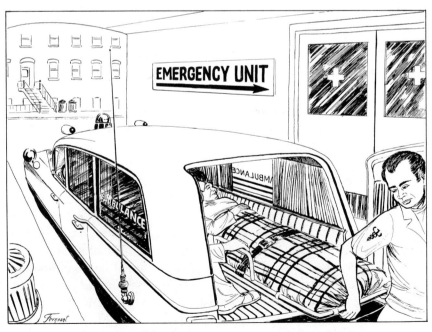

A patient being brought to an emergency unit in an ambulance.

equipment in emergency units is always in a state of readiness, and private doctors often do not have all the equipment for diagnosis and treatment in their offices.

Emergency units are very special areas in the hospital. Most units operate on a 24-hour basis. The emergency patients who are brought to the emergency unit generally require immediate attention. Those who come by *ambulance* are moved directly into a fully equipped treatment room. This room is located near the hospital's laboratory, x-ray department, and other special facilities. Waiting rooms allow family and friends to be comfortable while patients are treated.

The drama of the emergency room contrasts with the calm of the outpatient clinic. In both, however, the hospital is serving the community by providing health care services for a variety of medical conditions.

Discussion

1. Does the demand for hospital beds exceed the supply?

2. Why are many hospitals developing outpatient or extended care facilities? What are the advantages of outpatient facilities?

3. What kind of patients use outpatient facilities?

4. Explain what it means to be ambulatory. Give some examples of patients who are ambulatory and others who are not.

5. What kinds of health problems do the elderly have that make outpatient facilities ideal for their use?

6. What are self-care patients? Give some examples.

7. What is progressive hospital care?

8. Do patients with psychiatric problems use extended care facilities?

9. Identify several other ways in which patients use outpatient facilities.

10. Why are people using emergency units in hospitals more and more?

11. Are most emergency units open 24 hours a day?

12. Where are patients taken who are brought to the emergency room by ambulance?

13. Where can family and friends wait when a patient is taken to the emergency room?

Review

A. Are the following statements true or false? Explain your answers.

1. Outpatient services are becoming more and more widespread.

2. Visiting a hospital as an outpatient is cheaper than being confined as an inpatient.

3. Children are among the greatest users of extended care facilities.

4. To be able to use a self-care center, a patient should be ambulatory.

5. Most older people do not use outpatient services because they cannot afford to pay for them.

6. Rehabilitation by occupational therapy includes the use of massage.

7. Emergency units usually operate around the clock.

8. An ambulance is a machine used in an emergency unit to administer oxygen.

9. Hospitals that have progressive health care programs encourage patients to return home as soon as possible.

10. Psychiatric patients are too sick to be treated on an outpatient basis.

B. You are at home in the evening with your elderly father when he suddenly collapses on the living room floor. Explain what you do.

C. Explain which hospital facilities each of the following patients would be most likely to use. Choose from among inpatient, outpatient, and emergency facilities.

1. Post-coronary patient.
2. Child with measles.
3. Victim of a car accident.
4. Woman with an appendicitis attack.
5. Pregnant woman.
6. Dental patient.
7. Elderly man with a heart attack.
8. Veteran with an amputated leg doing physical therapy.
9. Child who has swallowed poison.
10. Patient desiring plastic surgery on her face for cosmetic reasons.

NOTES

NOTES

NOTES